Guibson Da Silva Litaiff

Influence of the restorative material on a monolithic implant crown

Guibson Da Silva Litaiff

Influence of the restorative material on a monolithic implant crown

In silico analysis of stress distribution

ScienciaScripts

Imprint

Any brand names and product names mentioned in this book are subject to trademark, brand or patent protection and are trademarks or registered trademarks of their respective holders. The use of brand names, product names, common names, trade names, product descriptions etc. even without a particular marking in this work is in no way to be construed to mean that such names may be regarded as unrestricted in respect of trademark and brand protection legislation and could thus be used by anyone.

Cover image: www.ingimage.com

This book is a translation from the original published under ISBN 978-613-9-63280-0.

Publisher:
Sciencia Scripts
is a trademark of
Dodo Books Indian Ocean Ltd. and OmniScriptum S.R.L publishing group

120 High Road, East Finchley, London, N2 9ED, United Kingdom
Str. Armeneasca 28/1, office 1, Chisinau MD-2012, Republic of Moldova, Europe
Printed at: see last page
ISBN: 978-620-7-63867-3

I dedicate it to my family, my father Hadoniram Barbosa Litaiff and my mother Eliana Camargo da Silva Litaiff, and especially to my partner Diuliane Menezes.

ACKNOWLEDGEMENTS

To the Faculty of Dentistry and the São Leopoldo Mandic Dental Research Centre, in the person of the Director General, Prof. Dr. José Luiz Cintra Junqueira, and the Director of Postgraduate Studies, Research and Extension, Prof. Dr. Marcelo Henrique Napimoga.

To the Master's coordinator and advisor of this work, Prof Dr Milton Edson Miranda, for his competence and for all the knowledge shared. Thank you very much for your patience and availability!

To my classmates, who became great friends and work partners, and contributed greatly to my personal and professional development.

To all those who helped in any way to carry out this work.

Thank you very much!

"It's not about getting to the top of the world and knowing you've won, it's about climbing and feeling that the path **has made** you **stronger.**"

(Ana Vilela)

SUMMARY

The aim of this study was to evaluate the influence of the prosthetic crown material on the biomechanical performance of the stress distribution received by the abutment (universal trunnion), implant (Morse cone) and bone tissue (cortical and medullary) in the first molar region, using the finite element method (FEM). Three three-dimensional in silico models representing the posterior region of the mandible were modelled using SolidWorks Professional 2013® software. Three different monolithic ceramic system materials were analysed for CAD/CAM (Computer *Aided Design/Computer Aided Manufacturing)* represented by models: DL - lithium disilicate, RN - nano ceramic resin and CP - polymer infiltrated ceramic. The modelled assembly was exported to Ansys Workbench 15.0® *software* to generate the three-dimensional mesh of quadratic finite elements. The FEM analysis was carried out to measure and evaluate the distribution of compressive stress in cortical and medullary bone, the quantitative and qualitative Von Mises stress in the implants and *abutments*, and tensile stress in the prosthetic crowns. The virtual models of the prosthetic crowns received occlusal compressive loading at 5 vertical points of 200N, relative to a physiological bite force in the first molar region. The results obtained were compared and the highest stress values were for the RN, cortical and medullary bone, implant and *abutment,* followed by the CP results, and with the lowest DL values. In the crown, the highest values were for DL, with average values for CP and the lowest values for the RN model. It can be concluded that the material of the crown influences the distribution of stresses and, according to the results, the DL model showed better biomechanical behaviour.

Keywords: Dental prosthesis. Dental Implant. Finite Element Analysis.

DISSEMINATION AND TRANSFER OF KNOWLEDGE

The aim of this study was to analyse the influence of the dental ceramic restoration material on the distribution of stresses generated by chewing in a posterior implant prosthesis using a 3D computer system. Three different ceramic materials were used, based on lithium disilicate, resin and polymers. The results obtained were compared and the highest stress values presented in cortical and medullary bone, implant and implant component were for nano-ceramic resin, followed by polymer-infiltrated ceramic and with the lowest results lithium disilicate. Therefore, it can be concluded that the crown material influences the biomechanics of stresses in implant prostheses and according to the results, lithium disilicate showed the best results compared to the other materials analysed.

SUMMARY

CHAPTER 1

INTRODUCTION

In dentistry, aesthetics has increased the search for restorative materials that provide better aesthetic and functional integration and biocompatibility between teeth and soft tissues. Currently, dental ceramics are the ones that best reproduce the physical properties of compressive strength, thermal conductivity, radiopacity, marginal integrity and colour stability, the optical characteristics of enamel and dentin, such as fluorescence, opalescence and translucency, and the ability to reproduce individualised textures and shapes (Guerra et al., 2007; Renzetti et al., 2013; Chen et al., 2014).

According to Deany (1996), metal-ceramic prostheses are currently being replaced by metal-free prostheses. Despite their excellent characteristics, metal-free prostheses have a high failure rate in the posterior region, regardless of whether they are ceramic or resin prostheses (Alshehri, 2011).

The CAD/CAM (Computer Aided Design/Computer Aided Manufacturing) system was developed in an attempt to facilitate the manufacture, reduce time and improve the mechanical properties of materials used to make indirect use restorations (El-Damanhoury et al., 2015). The use of this system is able to reduce failures and cracks in prostheses compared to the classic laboratory process (Tinschert et al., 2000; Beuer et al., 2008; Otto, Schneider, 2008).

Technical developments in the field of digital dentistry have opened up the opportunity to manufacture dental reconstructions using high-performance materials. In particular, monolithic ceramic materials (monoblocks or single layer ceramics), which are increasingly used to fabricate crowns for the restoration of natural teeth. These materials have addressed concerns about better fracture resistance properties compared to restorations with infrastructure materials covered by a veneering ceramic (Joda et al., 2015; Weyhrauch et al., 2016).

These materials can also be suitable for prosthetic restorations placed on implant abutments, characterising an alternative for implant-supported rehabilitations (Weyhrauch et al., 2016). Numerous restorative ceramic materials are used for CAD/CAM system technology, ranging from low to high hardness ceramic materials, such as lithium disilicate glass ceramics, and the more recently introduced hybrid ceramics, such as nano ceramic resin and polymer infiltrated ceramics (El-Damanhoury et al., 2015).

Lithium disilicate ceramics have a variety of colour shades and favourable translucency. It also has a high flexural strength of 360 MPa (Bindl et al., 2006). It is indicated for making inlays, onlays, ceramic laminates, anterior and posterior single crowns and fixed prostheses of up to three elements up to the second premolar (Giordano, 2006). According to Bindl et al. (2006), monolithic lithium disilicate ceramic prostheses have a high success rate and due to its properties, this material can also be successfully used in posterior implant prostheses.

According to its composition, nano ceramic resin (NCR) is classified as a composite resin, but its unique characteristics of durability, function and less crack propagation compared to glass ceramics classify it as a hybrid ceramic. In addition, RNC has a higher fracture resistance for non-retentive occlusal prostheses in posterior teeth when compared to some CAD/CAM ceramics (Magne et al., 2010). It has a lower flexural strength compared to lithium disilicate of 204 MPa and a modulus of elasticity (12.8 GPa) close to that of dentin, which would allow it to better absorb masticatory loads (Kassem et al., 2012; Chen et al., 2014; Joda et al., 2015). Therefore, in prostheses on implants in the posterior region, this property becomes quite interesting, since the material could better distribute the stresses that will be applied to the implant (Chen et al., 2014).

Polymer-infiltrated ceramic is a composite system that combines the properties of a ceramic matrix infiltrated by a polymeric structure, and can be classified as a hybrid ceramic. With a lower flexural strength compared to RNC, at approximately 160 MPa, its unique composition suggests a greater capacity to withstand mechanical loads by experiencing more elastic deformation before failure. This material is suitable for restorations of anterior and posterior full coverage single crowns, onlays, inlays and even laminated veneers (Kok et al., 2015; Rosentritt et al., 2017).

Most failures of implant-supported restorations occur after the installation of the crown which, added to occlusal forces, are subjected to stresses that can cause bone loss and shorten the lifespan of osseointegrated implants or increase the risk of prosthetic complications, such as ceramic fracture, crown decay, component fracture and others (Bayraktar et al., 2013).

Therefore, this study evaluated the influence of the prosthetic crown material on the biomechanical performance of the distribution of stresses received by the abutment, cone morse implants and bone tissue, when using three different monolithic ceramic systems for CAD/CAM, made from lithium disilicate ceramic, nano ceramic resin and polymer-infiltrated ceramic, in a lower first molar region, from the point of view of the three-dimensional finite element analysis method.

CHAPTER 2

LITERATURE REVIEW

2.1 Dental ceramics

Historically, ceramics were used as a dental material for the first time in 1774 in the manufacture of teeth for full dentures, by chemist Alexis Duchateau and dentist Nicholas Dubois. In 1886, by Land, dental ceramics were used for the first time as an indirect restorative material. Years later, with the invention of the electric furnace, new ways of handling ceramics were developed and patented, and the making of all-ceramic crowns on a platinum blade was realised in 1894, while low-fusion porcelains were developed in 1898. From 1903, ceramics entered the field of restorative dentistry with the use of porcelain jacket crowns (Kelly, Benetti, 2011; Mattei et al., 2011; Amoroso et al., 2012).

In 1956, Brecker introduced the metal-ceramic crown, combining auric alloys with porcelain, combining the aesthetics of cover ceramics with the mechanical resistance of metal infrastructure. This restorative material, which is still used today, has had its infrastructure modified by alternative alloys such as nickel-chromium and silver-palladium, and is indicated for restorations for posterior teeth, although its disadvantages include the presence of a cervical metal band, opacity in the presence of light and poor translucency (Guerra et al., 2007; Gomes et al., 2008; Mesquita, Vasques, 2016).

Feldspathic ceramics were the first to be manufactured in high fusion, where they were combined with metallic infrastructure alloys to form metal-ceramic crowns. These ceramics have excellent properties such as translucency, chemical stability, biocompatibility, resistance to compression and abrasion. However, due to their low mechanical strength and high fracture rate, their indication has been limited to anterior single crowns, as has their use as a pure feldspathic crown (Kramer et al., 2009). The use of feldspathic ceramics in posterior teeth and fixed partial dentures has become possible thanks to the association of porcelain with metal as a covering material, providing resistance to fracture and marginal adequacy (Rolim et al., 2013).

In order for ceramics to be used without a metal structure, various crystals were added to the crystalline phase, thus increasing the physical characteristics of this material, to the detriment of its glassy phase, which is responsible for its translucency (Marson et al., 2013). In order to improve its mechanical strength, in 1965, Mclean and Hughes developed the first feldspathic ceramic reinforced with aluminium oxide. Since 1990, feldspathic ceramics have been associated with leucite crystals as a modifying agent, in high concentrations of 40% to 50% by weight, and are now indicated for anterior and posterior single crowns, laminated veneer restorations, inlays and onlays, although they still have a low flexural strength of around 180 MPa (Garcia et al., 2011; Mattei et al., 2011; Amoroso et al., 2012; Rolim et al., 2013). The addition of lithium disilicate crystals dispersed in a glassy matrix has improved the mechanical properties of feldspathic ceramics without, however, compromising their optical properties (Bindl et al., 2006; Bispo, 2015).

2.1.1 Lithium disilicate

The first description of the use of lithium disilicate ceramics was by Brodkin in 1998, by means of temperature pressing. In 1999, it was used as an infrastructure associated with veneering ceramics (Zandinejad et al., 2015). Lithium disilicate ceramic, whether processed by milling or high-temperature pressing, was initially developed as an infrastructure material that provided greater translucency than other high strength ceramic systems, but it has been used more as a single restorative material, i.e. monolithic, for full crowns (Silva et al., 2012).

Lithium disilicate ceramic material for use in all-ceramic restorations is available in monolithic ceramic blocks, which are milled using CAD/CAM technology. This material has a high crystalline concentration of lithium disilicate of around 70% by volume in a glassy matrix. The crystallisation of this material takes place in a two-stage process. Initially it has 40% precipitated lithium metasilicate crystals in its volume with crystals of 0.2 to 1.0 pm, resulting in a violet-blue block. The final crystallisation takes place through vacuum heating at 850°C, which results in a ceramic with a high crystalline content of fine lithium disilicate crystals of approximately 1.5 pm, incorporated into a glassy matrix in the colour of the selected tooth (Fasbinder et al., 2010; Badawy et al., 2016).

The development of this system resulted in improvements in the physical properties of ceramics, with high flexural strength (360 MPa), modulus of elasticity (95 Gpa) and Poisson's ratio of 0.30 (Silva et al., 2012; Chen et al., 2014; Rosentritt et al., 2017). These ceramics have made it possible to make inlays, onlays, overlays, single crowns and laminate veneers, and are now also indicated for crowns on posterior teeth and implants (Fasbinder et al., 2010). Lithium disilicate has excellent aesthetic characteristics, which can be advantageous in restorations on implants, which require high fracture resistance and balanced aesthetics (Poticny, Klim, 2010).

2.2 Hybrid ceramics

One of the main objectives of restorative dentistry is to replace the lost tooth structure with a material whose structure and physical properties are similar to a natural tooth. Ceramics, due to their chemical stability, have good mechanical and optical properties. However, once placed in the mouth, its repair, if necessary, is problematic. Most ceramics are considered fragile due to their high modulus of elasticity and low fracture resistance, often due to cracks within the restorative material (Al-Makramani et al., 2011; Albero et al., 2015).

In order to obtain a material with better physical properties, various materials have been introduced to the market, such as those based on resin composites in blocks for the CAD/CAM system, which combine the modulus of elasticity of resin composites similar to that of dentin and characteristics of glass ceramics similar to enamel, adding aesthetics and durability. These materials are represented by nano-ceramic resin and polymer-infiltrated ceramics (Lim et al., 2016). Although they are of the same material class, they are manufactured in different ways and have different performance (Badawy et al., 2016).

2.2.1 Nano ceramic resin

In order to solve the difficulties of other materials, both aesthetically and functionally and the propagation of cracks, a new type of material has been developed, belonging to the RNC category of composites (Chen et al., 2014; Awada & Nathanson, 2015). The system represented in a monolithic block is based on a nanotechnology consisting of both nanometric particles and nanoagglomerates with a total nanoceramic material content of approximately 80 per cent by weight, incorporated into a highly crosslinked resin matrix of 20 per cent (El-Damanhoury et al., 2015; Cekic-Nagas et al., 2016). One of the main characteristics of this material is its microstructure, specifically composed of monodisperse silica nanoparticles 20 nm in diameter and zirconia 4 and 11 nm in diameter, as well as zirconia-silica nanoagglomerates of 0.6 to 10 pm (Lim et al., 2016; Badawy et al., 2016).

This particle size distribution gives the material excellent characteristics, combining polish retention and optical properties with high wear resistance and mechanical properties close to the natural tooth, showing flexural strength (204 MPa), modulus of elasticity (12.8 Gpa) and Poisson's ratio of 0.3 (Chen et al., 2014; Joda et al., 2015). Nano-ceramic resin is indicated for single-unit full crown restorations, inlay, onlay, laminate veneers, and especially implant prostheses, as it is supposed to be able to absorb small masticatory stresses, be resilient and non-fragile (Awada & Nathanson, 2015; Dogan et al., 2017).

2.2.2 Polymer-infiltrated ceramics

Another monolithic hybrid system of restorative materials for CAD/CAM is polymer-infiltrated ceramic, which consists of a ceramic matrix with a sintered structure, the pores of which are filled with a polymeric material after the application of a bonding agent. The mass percentage of the inorganic ceramic is 86% by weight and 14% of the organic polymer part, made up of UDMA (urethane dimethacrylate) and TEGDMA (triethylene glycol dimethacrylate). Its ceramic composition corresponds to a fine feldspathic ceramic structure enriched with aluminium oxide (Kok et al., 2015; Badawy et al., 2016; Cekic-Nagas et al., 2016; Zhi et al., 2016).

The combination of these materials provides excellent benefits, such as a lower tendency to crack when compared to pure ceramics, as well as increasing the ability to withstand mechanical loading, presenting more elastic deformation before failure. It has a modulus of elasticity of 37.95 GPa, flexural strength of 160 MPa and Poisson's ratio of 0.23 (Della Bona et al., 2014; Rosentritt et al., 2017). Polymer-infiltrated ceramics can be used for definitive single-tooth restorations for full crowns, inlays, onlays, veneers and implant-supported crowns. Its hardness values and modulus of elasticity similar to those of dental tissues make this material a good choice for restorations in anterior and posterior areas (Albero et al., 2015).

2.3 Finite element method

The finite element method is a mathematical method for analysing the performance and deformation of structures of any geometry, in which the continuous medium is discretised into small elements, in a given (finite) quantity. This methodology makes it possible to model complex structures with irregular geometries, such as natural and artificial fabrics, and to modify the parameters of their geometry. This makes it possible to apply a system of forces at any point and/or direction, thus providing information on the displacement and degree of tension caused by these loads to the dental element or tissue being analysed. The in silico study of the effect of loads applied to teeth or implants is of great scientific interest and involves a variety of methodologies (Lotti et al., 2006; Trivedi, 2014).

The development of FEM had its origins at the end of the 18th century, but it was only later, with the advent of computing, that this analysis became more practical. In 1960, Turner, Clough, Martins and Topp used the name finite element method for the first time, based on work on a previous aircraft project, in which they proposed an analysis method similar to the FEM (Lotti et al., 2006).

The FEM has been used for some time in experiments related to dentistry, in various specialities. The pioneers in the use of FEM in implant dentistry were Weinstein in 1976, an area for which it would prove to be of great importance in biomechanics studies (Geng et al., 2001). In Brazil, the first research using FEM in dentistry was presented by Corrêa & Matson in 1977, who demonstrated the superiority of this method compared to photoelasticity. Blatt et al. (2006) also reported on the complexity and limitations of the photoelastic method, whose numerical results could easily be obtained using FEM.

Assessing the biomechanical performance of implant-supported rehabilitations has certain limitations, which makes it interesting to use alternative methodologies to carry out this assessment. Analysing the biomechanical performance of implant-supported rehabilitations is directly associated with analysing the stresses on implants, bone (cortical and medullary) and prosthetic components. The most commonly used methodologies for analysing stresses in the peri-implant region are photoelasticity, extensometry and finite elements (Takahashi, 2011; Bayraktar et al., 2013).

Trivedi (2014) and Lee et al. (2017) cited the widespread acceptance of FEM as a non-invasive and excellent tool for studying biomechanics and the influence of mechanical forces on biological systems, since, with advances in digital imaging systems, computed tomography (CT) and magnetic resonance imaging (MRI), it has become possible to determine individual specific data on the geometry and properties of bone for FEM modelling, making it possible to develop structures such as cortical bone, medullary bone, implants and prosthetic components, at the micro level and in three dimensions. Thus, more accurate anatomical models could be created, which in turn would provide more reliable results.

According to Moraes et al. (2013), the physical properties of titanium and metal alloys generally vary little. This is not the case with the properties of cortical and medullary bone, which can vary from patient to patient, or according to age and region (maxilla or mandible). Approximate values found in the literature are used for the analyses. It is common for all the materials involved to be considered homogeneous and isotropic, where the material's properties are the same in all directions. On the other hand, it is known that both cortical and medullary bone are not homogeneous and therefore have variations in modulus of elasticity depending on the region. Similarly, the bone/implant interface is considered to be homogeneous and continuous across the entire surface of the implant, which is not necessarily true.

Despite the inherent limitations of simulating an in silico study, in which clinical situations may not be fully reproduced, experimental techniques on humans and animals are also limited due to the variability of factors that can lead to errors when applying complex force systems to living beings (Lotti et al., 2006). Trivedi (2014) emphasised that finite elements have several advantages compared to studies on real models. The experiments can be replicated and modulated in a desirable way, and there are few ethical considerations for the study. Takahashi (2011) cited FEM as an attractive method because of the similarities that can be reproduced between finite element models and real clinical situations, due to the possibility of simulating cortical and medullary bone structures, as well as the geometries of implants and prosthetic components, and the application of dynamic loading. Moraes et al. (2013) highlighted this methodology as complementary to clinical studies, revealing additional information on biomechanics and stress distribution in implant-supported rehabilitations.

According to Geng et al. (2001), when making finite element models, certain assumptions must be made that can influence the results obtained after analysis. Some of these assumptions relate to the detail of the bone and implant geometry to be modelled, the properties of the materials and the boundary and interface conditions between bone and implant.

The first step in obtaining an experimental model in FEM is to model the geometry of the structure on the computer, which is drawn graphically in a specific computer program. Subsequently, the modelled structure is discretised into small elements that represent coordinates in space and can take different shapes, such as tetrahedral or hexahedral, where the greater the number of elements, the more accurate the models. At the ends of each finite element are the nodes, which connect the elements to each other, forming a mesh arranged in two or three-dimensional layers. Each node has a defined number of degrees of freedom, which characterise how the node will move in space. This displacement can be described in three spatial dimensions (X, Y and Z) (Geng et al., 2001; Lotti et al., 2006; Gultekin et al., 2012).

Blatt et al. (2006) stated that the properties of materials have a great influence on the stresses and distribution of tensions in a structure. In FEM these properties can be modelled as isotropic and anisotropic (orthotropic), where in an isotropic material its mechanical performance is the same in all directions and in an anisotropic material it has different properties when measured in different directions. In most studies, biological materials and structures are assumed to be homogeneous, linearly elastic and isotropic, characterised by two material constants: **Young's modulus of elasticity (E),** which represents the slope of the linear stress/strain portion of the material, and **Poisson's** ratio **(v), which** refers to the absolute value of the ratio between transverse and longitudinal deformations in an axial traction axis.

The transmission of loads and the resulting distribution of stresses at the bone-implant interface should be the goal of finite element analysis. Once the properties have been determined, the necessary loads are applied and the results are analysed, representing the distribution of stresses and deformations in the model. The results are displayed using a colour scale, where each shade corresponds to an amount of displacement or stress generated in the structures or any other object of analysis in the three directions of space (X, Y and Z) (Geng et al., 2001; Lotti et al., 2006, Gultekin et al., 2012).

2.4 Stress distribution in implant-supported restorations

Implant-supported restorations have been widely used for rehabilitations in edentulous areas as a treatment with good clinical prospects and a reliable method. The success rate of implants is based on osseointegration, which, together with the prosthetic restoration, determines the survival rate. There are two types of failure: early complications, which occur before prosthetics, mainly due to tissue inflammation, and late complications after osseointegration and restoration, due to bone resorption around the dental implant. This means that all successful implants still carry the risk of late failures, which are related to the longevity and quality of the treatment. Under physiological functional loading conditions, bone loss of 1 to 1.5 mm can be expected over the first year and less than 0.2 mm each year thereafter. Therefore, biomechanical factors should be widely considered when planning implant-supported rehabilitations, due to their main responsibility for bone resorption. This process can be accelerated by chemical, mechanical and biological factors (Kitamura et al., 2004; Maminskas et al., 2016).

Several mechanical and biological factors can be considered as possible etiologies of early bone loss around dental implants, such as surgical trauma, occlusal overload, peri-implantitis, presence of micro-mismatches, material properties, implant-abutment design, among others (Geng et al., 2001; Menini et al., 2013). Mechanical loading associated with implant-abutment design or prosthetic geometry plays an important role in long-term success from the moment of initial implant loading. However, occlusal loading during chewing is distributed through the prosthetic materials and the implant to the peri-implant bone (Macedo et al., 2017). In addition, Geng et al. (2001) and Takahashi (2011) cited that the transfer of occlusal load between the bone/implant interface depends not only on the occlusal load, but also on the material in which the prosthesis is manufactured, the nature of the bone/implant interface, bone quantity and quality and the geometry of the implant selected (length, diameter and shape).

Merz et al. (2000) reported that the implant-abutment connection system also potentially affects the distribution of stresses in prosthetic components, bone tissue and prostheses. Various abutment connection systems have been devised, external and internal hexagonal connections, and conical joint systems with a conical or Morse cone seal, the latter presenting some advantages over the others, added to better joint sealing. Conical joint connections are more stable and resistant than other connections and are also more difficult to release. In addition, Kitamura et al. (2004) reported that conical interface connections promote a reduction in stress distribution compared to butt joints.

Occlusal overload is considered one of the risk factors for implant longevity. Geng et al. (2001) stated that in order to maintain bone health, loads of between 1.4 and 5 MPa are necessary;

any values outside this threshold can be considered overloads. A healthy tooth surrounded by periodontal ligament has 25 to 100 pm of micromovements in the axial axis. In comparison, an osseointegrated implant can move only 3 to 5 pm in the same axis, which is determined by the deformation of the bone (Pita et al., 2008; Maminskas et al., 2016). Thus, the biomechanics of the transfer and distribution of stresses applied to the implant-crown system occurs through a rigid and direct interface, whereby any force applied to the implant-crown system is transferred directly to the bone. Mechanical tension plays an eminent role in maintaining bone homeostasis, where occlusal overload is a predisposing factor for the risk of peri-implant bone loss (Macedo et al., 2017).

In implant dentistry, not only axial or horizontal forces should be considered, but the combination of both that reflect the clinical applicability of the condition, determining a more real characteristic of the occlusion (Von Mises) (Pita et al., 2008). Studies such as that by Chen et al. (2014), which evaluated static axial loads, concluded that the greatest variations in stress values occurred when the modulus of elasticity of the materials was altered, specifically with regard to the restorative material. According to the studies by Menini et al. (2013), the use of different restorative materials in implant-supported rehabilitations affects the distribution of stresses in the peri-implant region, emphasising that more resilient materials reduced the values found. Skalak (1983) mentioned that viscoelastic materials, such as acrylic resin, for restorative material, delay and reduce the transmission of forces compared to materials with a high modulus of elasticity.

However, several studies have refuted the existence of the shock absorption capacity of resilient materials (Menini et al., 2013). The effect of the restorative material of the prosthesis is still controversial, however, a consensus is that the properties of the implant material increase the effect and location of stress concentrations at the bone-implant interface (Geng et al., 2001).

Stresses of various types are used to assess mechanical stresses in peri-implant bone tissue, including Von Mises stress, minimum principal stress (compression) and maximum principal stress (tension), and shear stress. The Von Mises stress is the most frequently used, mainly to evaluate stresses and the performance of various materials (Triveti, 2014). As described by Silva (2005), the

Von Mises criterion, or maximum distortion energy theory, is of particular importance when considering the maximum resistance of a structure when subjected to two states of stress (tension and compression). This criterion is based on determining the distortion energy of the structure, i.e. the energy related to changes in its shape, as opposed to the energy linked to changes in its volume.

The FEM makes it possible to simulate the stress distribution area of the occlusal load for the implant, cortical bone and medullary bone, from the cervical region to the apex of the implants. The simulations predict problems in the prosthesis-implant connection, failures in the retention screw and other prosthetic components and even in the restorative material, even before they are tested in vivo. These investigations highlight the importance of analysing the biomechanical condition of the implant-bone interface for the long-term success of implants (Macedo et al., 2017).

CHAPTER 3

PROPOSAL

21

The purpose of this in silico study was to evaluate and compare the influence of the type of monolithic ceramic used in the prosthetic crown, using lithium disilicate, nano-ceramic resin and polymer-infiltrated ceramic, in terms of the biomechanical performance of stress distribution in abutments, implants and peri-implant bone tissue, with the hypothesis that materials with lower elastic modulus (RNC) values would perform better in terms of stress distribution in posterior implant-supported rehabilitations.

CHAPTER 4

MATERIAL AND METHOD

4.1 Ethical aspects

The study in question received full exemption from the São Leopoldo Mandic Faculty's Research Ethics Committee on 7th May 2015, as it was a laboratory study with no involvement of human beings or materials derived from them, and is included in Annex A of this paper.

4.2 Experimental design

Three three-dimensional finite element analysis models representing the posterior region of the mandible were designed, in a point-by-point mesh, containing cortical and medullary bone characteristics, all with equal dimensions. Titanium implants with a Morse cone platform and abutments for a cemented crown, also in titanium, were positioned on the models.

Single implant-supported crowns simulating rehabilitation in the posterior region of the mandible, relating to the 1st molar, were designed by varying only the type of prosthetic crown material (figure 1). A force of 200N was applied to this assembly at five occlusal points with axial loading, verifying the distribution of these loads to the cortical bone, medullary bone, implant and abutment.

The materials and methods adopted in this study are separated into topics, covering the modelling conditions and computer support used, mathematical analyses of the finite element method, loading and stress criteria. This method allows the researcher to predict how these stresses are distributed in the contact areas of the implant, abutment and prosthetic crown around the cortical bone and medullary bone, and can be defined to obtain the solution of a complex mechanical system.

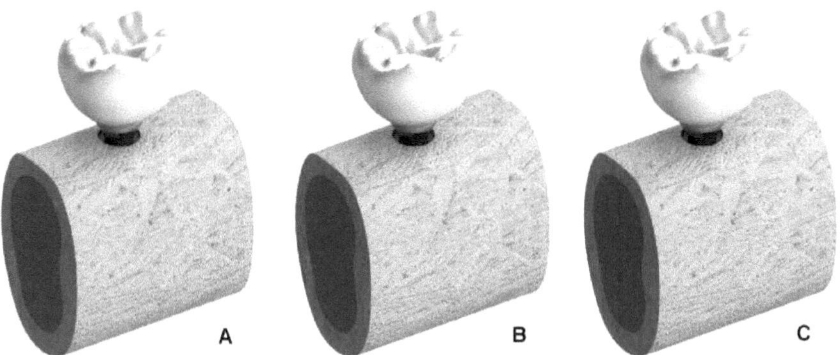

Figure 1 - Illustration of the three FEM models.
Legend: Models A) lithium disilicate; B) nano-ceramic resin; C) polymer-infiltrated ceramic.

Source: Own authorship.

4.3 Modelling parts

The virtual construction of three 3D (three-dimensional) models was carried out using software for three-dimensional modelling by assisted drawing (figure 2), in this case SolidWorks Professional 2013® (3Dtech-Solidworks, São Paulo, SP, Brazil), to assess the distribution of stresses when using different monolithic crown materials.

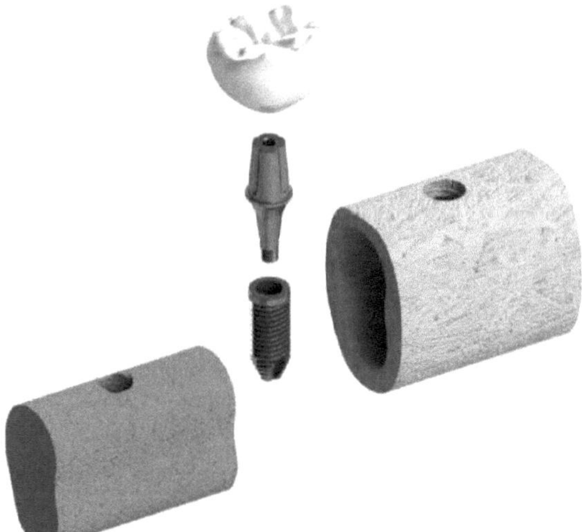

Figure 2 - Illustration of three-dimensional modelling

Source: Own authorship.

4.3.   1 Bone tissue

A representative piece of bone tissue in the posterior region of the mandible was modelled based on the mandibular dimensions and contours, with a cortical thickness of 1.5 mm and medullary bone height compatible with the installation of an implant. The model was made up of two individual pieces of cortical and medullary bone tissue, so that it was possible to discriminate the properties (modulus of elasticity and Poisson's ratio) of each type of bone. Once the structure had been contoured, a 10 mm-long bone block was removed horizontally so that components could be attached without interfering with the distribution of stresses (figure 3).

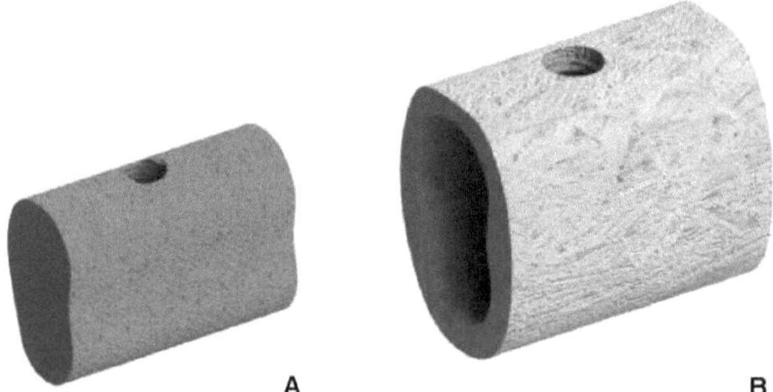

Figure 3 - Illustration of the modelled bone tissue.
Legend: A) Medullary bone; B) Cortical bone.

Source: Own authorship.

4.3.   2 Implant

The dimensions and geometry of the implant were based on commercially available products and did not represent a specific company. A Morse cone platform implant, with a height of 11 mm and a width of 4.0 mm, was modelled together with a universal abutment for cemented crowns, with a height of 6 mm, a diameter of 4.5 mm and a transmucosal of 2.5 mm (figure 4).

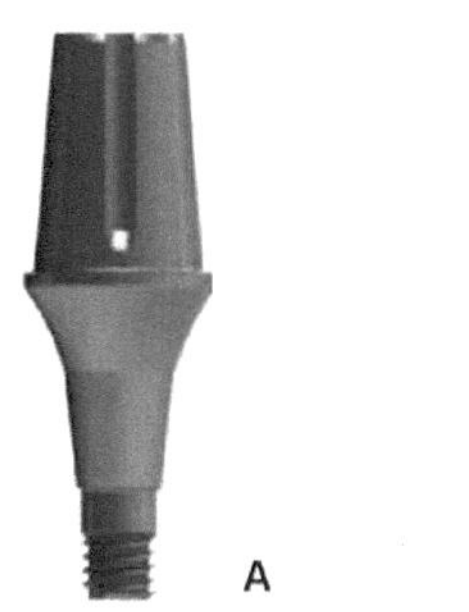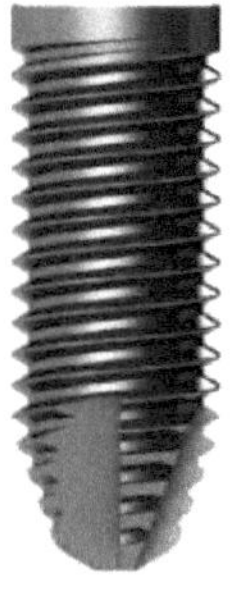

Figure 4 - Illustration of the abutment and modelled Morse cone implant.

Caption: A) Morse cone abutment for cemented crowns; B) Morse cone implant. Source: Author.

4.3.3 Prosthetic crown

The factors under study consisted of the influence of different types of implant-supported prosthetic crown materials on the biomechanical performance of stress distribution, simulated by three different monolithic ceramic systems. For the prosthetic rehabilitation simulations, three representative prosthetic crown pieces were constructed, which were modelled following the anatomical references of the average size of a human lower first molar, with 11 mm in the mesiodistal direction, 10.5 mm in the buccal-lingual direction, and a central fossa depth of 1.5 mm (figure 5) (Kim et al., 2013; Bindl et al., 2006).

After modelling, the crown was positioned concentrically (central axis aligned) to the central axis of the implant. Three three-dimensional in silico models of implant-supported crowns with different monolithic ceramic systems were developed, represented by:

DL model: lithium disilicate

RN model: nano ceramic resin

CP model: polymer-infiltrated ceramic

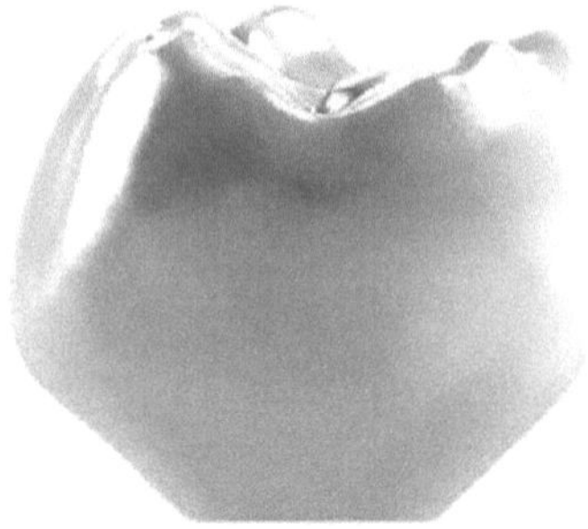

Figure 5 - Illustration of the modelled prosthetic crown.

Source: Own authorship.

4.4   Finite element analysis

The virtual models were positioned on a representative model of a posterior mandibular section, composed of cortical and medullary bone. The modelled set (IGES format) was exported to Ansys Workbench 14.0 software (Swanson Analysis Systems, Canonsburg, Philadelphia, United States) to generate the 3D mesh of finite quadratic elements with a size of 0.7 mm, defined after convergence analysis at 5% (figures 6 and 7).

The convergence analysis aims to determine the element size to be used during the analysis. To do this, the mesh was successively refined (reducing the size of the element) and tested in terms of the application of loads and the interpretation of stress values. Convergence was reached when the difference between the stress of a given mesh and the subsequent (more refined) mesh was less than 5%. Table 1 shows the number of nodes and elements that made up each model.

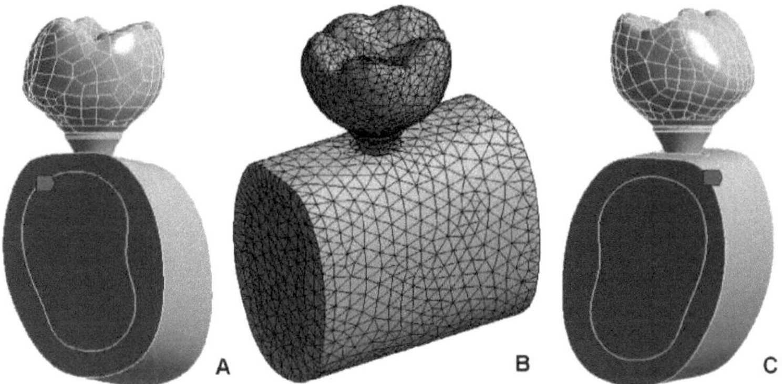

Figure 6 - Mesh generated with 0.7 mm tetrahedral elements.
Caption: A) and C) Lateral views of the fixation of the crown model to the cortical bone; B) Front view of the generated mesh.

Source: Own authorship.

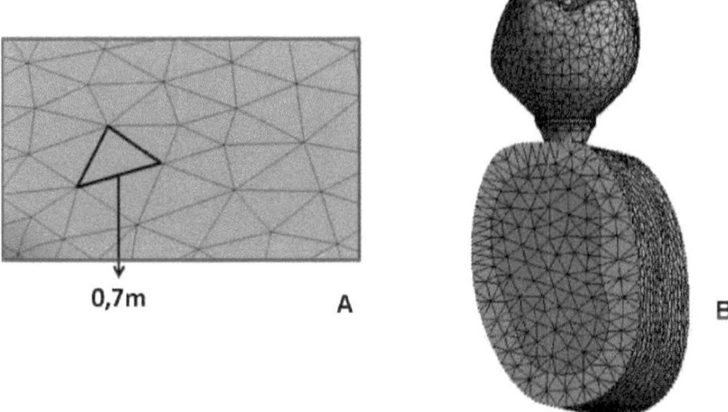

Figure 7 - Side view of the mesh emphasising the 0.7 mm tetrahedral elements.
Legend: A) Detail of the element at 0.7 mm; B) Side view of the point-to-point model.

Source: Own authorship.

Table 1 - Composition of the models generated.

MODELS	WE	ELEMENTS
LITHIUM DISILICATE	118.391	69.020
NANO CERAMIC RESIN	118.391	69.020
POLYMER-INFILTRATED CERAMICS	118.391	69.020

Source: Own authorship.

FEM analysis was carried out to measure and evaluate the distribution of compressive stresses in cortical and medullary bone, the quantitative and qualitative Von Mises stress in implants and abutments, and the maximum tensile stress in prosthetic crowns, evaluating the distribution of these loads in silico. The models were considered homogeneous, isotropic and linearly elastic. To feed the software and characterise the performance of the materials, the mechanical properties of Young's Modulus (GPa) and Poisson's Ratio (V) were used, based on data available in the literature (table 2).

Table 2 - Properties of the simulated models.

MATERIAL	YOUNG MODULUS (GPa)	POISSON'S RATIO (V)	REFERENCES
CORTICAL BONE	13,7	0,30	Cruz et al. (2009)
MEDULLARY BONE	1,37	0,30	Cruz et al. (2009)
TITANIUM	110,0	0,33	Cruz et al. (2009)
LITHIUM DISILICATE	95,0	0,30	Chen et al. (2014)
NANO CERAMIC RESIN	12,8	0,30	Chen et al. (2014)
POLYMER-INFILTRATED CERAMICS	30,0	0,23	Lim et al. (2016)

Source: Own authorship.

4.4.1 Loading

The models were subjected to occlusal loading on the crown surface of the implant-supported teeth, simulating masticatory force in the posterior mandible. A load of 200N was applied to the lower first molar, divided into five standardised points on the crown and evenly distributed on the centric cusp tip and bottom of the central fossa, longitudinal to the implant axis. All the models were loaded with the same characteristics (figure 8).

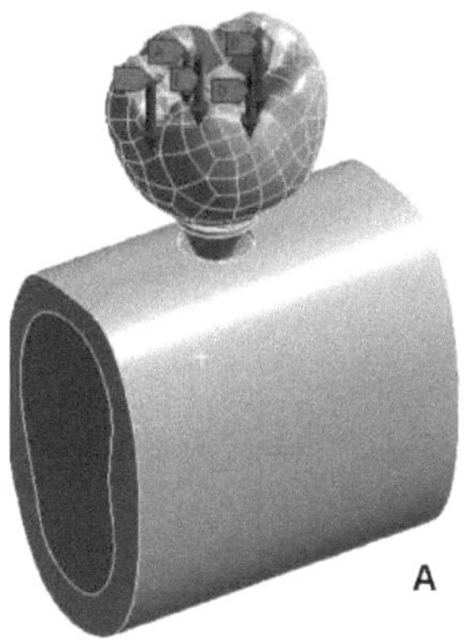 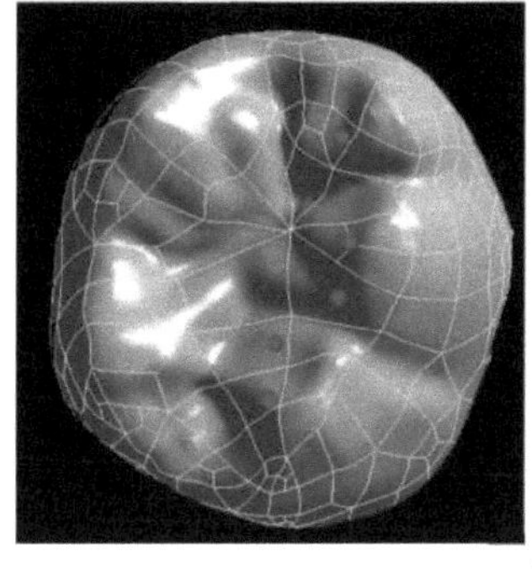

Figure 8 - Application of 200 N at 5 points on the occlusal surface.
Legend: A) 5 loading points; B) location of the occlusal points.

Source: Own authorship.

4.5 Analysing data

The stress values were analysed from the graphic images of the stresses using the Von Mises criterion (implant and abutment) and also by compression stress analysis (cortical bone and medullary bone). The quantitative analysis was carried out by distributing the colour gradient of the images, associated with the numerical scale, describing the maximum and minimum value of each colour, which represents the level of stress in a given region, in MPa (table 3). The qualitative analysis was carried out by distributing the colours in each model.

Table 3 - Criteria for finite element analysis.

COMPONENTS	CRITERIA
CROWN	Maximum principal stress (tensile)
ABUTMENT	Von Mises stress
IMPLANT	Von Mises stress
CORTICAL BONE	Minimum principal tension (compression)
MEDULLARY BONE	Minimum principal tension (compression)

Source: Own authorship.

CHAPTER 5

RESULTS

After analysing the data by quantitative and qualitative observation, the results were divided up to individually analyse the stress generated in each region: bone tissue (cortical and medullary), implants, abutment and prosthetic crowns. The quantitative data, in MPa, for all regions and components can be seen in Table 4.

Table 4 - Stress distribution according to model region, based on crown material variation in MPa.

REGION	DL	RN	CP
CROWN	28,45	28,16	28,40
ABUTMENT	60,14	65,53	63,08
IMPLANT	53,78	57,66	55,90
CORTICAL COMPRESSION	14,41	14,89	14,67
SPINAL CORD COMPRESSION	5,44	5,45	5,45

Source: Own authorship.

5.1 Stress distribution in bone tissue

The compression generated by applying the load to the bone tissue was greater in cortical bone than in medullary bone, regardless of the crown material used. For the cortical bone region, the model with the lowest minimum peak compressive stress was the DL model, which was lower than the others

models. The RN model showed the highest peak compressive stress in cortical bone, as shown in Graph 1.

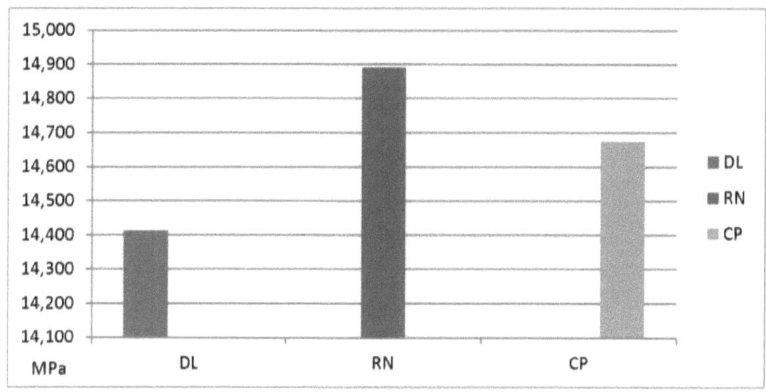

Graph 1 - Variation of values in peri-implant cortical bone tissue.

Source: Own authorship.

In all three models, the compressive stress peaks were located in the outermost bone region in contact with the first threads of the implant installed in the first molar area.

In the medullary bone, the tension peaks were localised in the region in contact with the implant apex in all models. The compression values in the medullary tissue were similar between the models. The distribution pattern of the three simulated models can be seen in Figures 9 and 10 respectively.

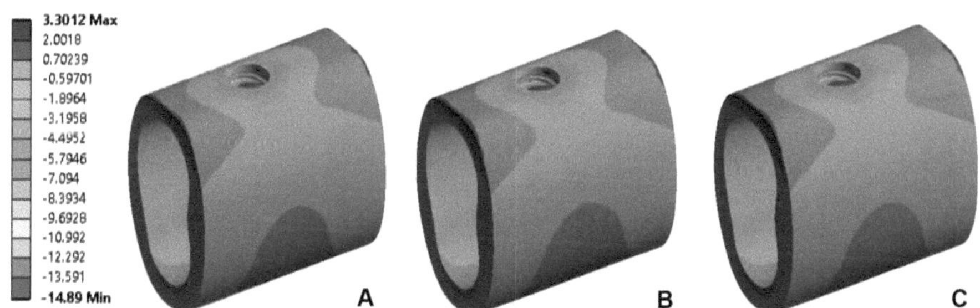

Figure 9 - Distribution of stresses from the implant to the cortical bone.
Legend: Models relating to: (A) DL; (B) RN; (C) CP.
Source: Own authorship.

31

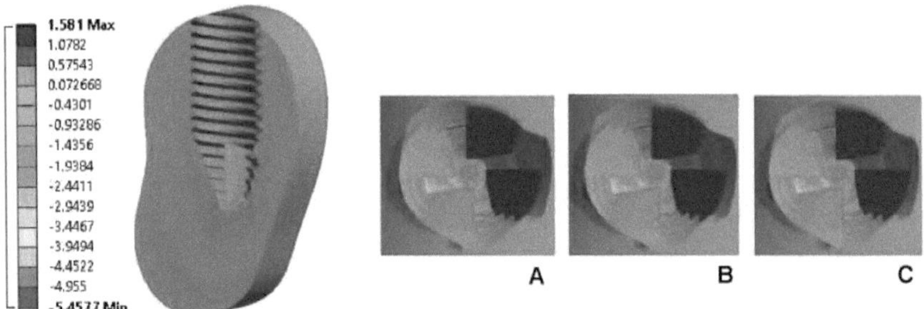

Figure 10 - Distribution of stresses from the implant to the medullary bone.
Legend: Models relating to: (A) DL; (B) RN; (C) CP.

Source: Own authorship.

5.   2Distribution of stresses in the implant

For the implants evaluated in the first molar region, there was a relative variation in the distribution of Von Mises stresses in the different simulated models according to the materials of the prosthetic crowns. The highest Von Mises stress peaks occurred in the RN model with a value of 57.66 MPa, shown in figure 11.

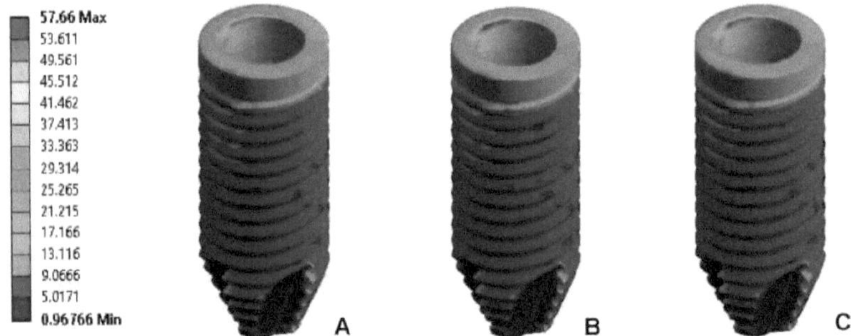

Figura 11   - Stresses on the inner edge of the implant.

Legend: A) DL; B) RN; C) CP.

Source: Own authorship.

5.   3 Stress distribution in the prosthetic abutment

Similarly to the evaluation described above, when analysing the stresses received in the abutment models evaluated, there was a variation in the distribution of Von Mises stresses according to the different materials of the prosthetic crowns. The highest Von Mises stress peaks occurred in the RN model with 65.53 MPa.

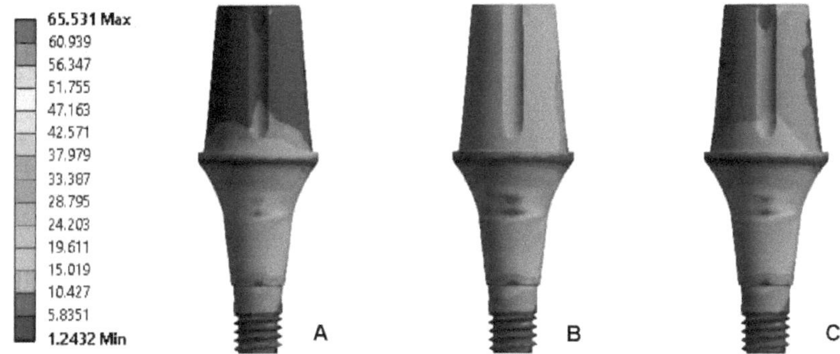

Figure 12 - Stresses in the prosthetic abutment joint.

Legend: A) DL; B) RN; C) CP.

Source: Own authorship.

Figure 12 shows the occurrence of Von Mises stress peaks in the prosthetic abutments, whose stresses were more prominent in the region of the joint in contact with the inner face of the implants.

5.   4Stress distribution   in the prosthetic crown

Alongside the implant and abutment models, the prosthetic crowns, which formed the variable in the study presented with anatomical characteristics and installed in the first molar region, were evaluated and there was a relative variation in the five points of the distribution of the maximum principal tensile stresses in the different simulated models, according to the different materials of the prosthetic crowns. Shown sequentially in figure 13. The data analysis showed small variations in the distribution of stresses between the models representing the ceramic crown materials. The most representative was the DL model with values of 28.45 MPa.

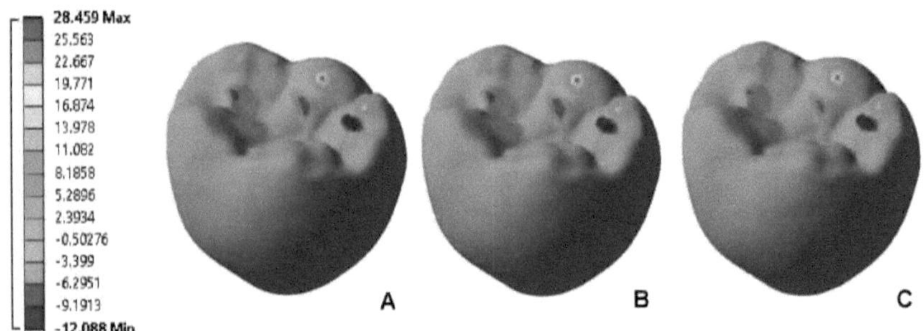

Figure 13 - Distribution of occlusal loads on the crowns.

Legend: A) DL; B) RN; C) CP.

Source: Own authorship.

CHAPTER 6

DISCUSSION

According to Menini et al. (2013), the resilience of the crown material influences the stress exerted on the implant. For these reasons, in the current study, occlusal loads were directed onto the occlusal surface of the crown, verifying the distribution of stresses by analysing the finite element method, what the variation in ceramic materials chosen for the crown means for shock absorption and how this could influence bone remodelling.

Taking into account studies such as Merz et al. (2000), for this research we chose to analyse rehabilitations with cone morse (CM) prosthetic interface implants, which have demonstrated superior mechanics and thus better long-term prosthetic stability when compared to implants with butt joints. In addition, Macedo et al. (2017) emphasise that the CM implant interface resists lateral loads, preventing the abutment threads from loosening, as well as being stable and free from rotation, which reduces the risk of mechanical complications such as loss or fracture of the abutment screw. In this study, crowns were used on Morse cone platform implants with a height of 11 mm and a width of 4.0 mm, and abutments with a height of 6 mm and a diameter of 4.5 mm, standardised for cemented prostheses according to studies by Joda et al. (2015) and Kim et al. (2013).

Research such as Bonfante et al. (2015), Weyhrauch et al. (2016) and Dogan et al. (2017) used monolithic implant crowns on a first molar in the mandible to assess the fracture resistance of the different materials used to make cemented crowns by subjecting them to universal testing machines, resulting in different failure modules for each material, thus simulating the basic element of a functional occlusion in the area of greatest concentration of occlusal load and stress. Kok et al. (2015), in their research using universal testing methodology and FEM, used crowns in the shape of lower first molars on abutments, and emphasised that it is in this region that implant-supported crowns are most likely to fail, both from cracks and fractures, as well as stress distribution when it exceeds a certain limit, which can lead to bone loss around the cervical region and ultimately the loss of the implant. For the current study, the standardised occlusal anatomy of the crowns was based on the methodology of Kim et al. (2013) and Rosentritt et al. (2017), in which the occlusal characteristics of a mandibular 1st molar, with 11 mm in the mesio-distal direction, 10.5 mm in the lingual vestibule direction, and a central fossa depth of 1.5 mm, allowed each specimen to be mounted in the same reproducible load position in contact with the equally distributed cusps (Dogan et al., 2017). As reproduced in this study, which simulates basic elements of a functional occlusion, therefore making it clinically relevant.

According to Joda et al. (2015), the CAD/CAM system is a promising option for manufacturing reconstructions with constant quality, associated with monolithic materials with high hardness, generating a streamlined workflow, especially in the functional zone of the posterior regions. These materials, according to the studies by Albero et al. (2015), Aboushelib & Elsafi (2016) and Badawy et al. (2016) were evaluated using universal testing machines for fracture resistance, varying only the monolithic materials of the crowns, from glass ceramics such as lithium disilicate to resin-modified hybrid ceramics such as nano ceramic resin and polymer-infiltrated ceramics, which were chemically and physically different, following the same pattern, all ceramic blocks milled using the CAD/CAM system.

Little research is available on the use of these materials and their properties in posterior crowns, in terms of stress distribution or shock absorption capacity, as represented in the studies by Chen et al. (2014) and Kok et al. (2015), who used the finite element method to analyse the biomechanical performance of these implant materials. These findings confirm the importance of carrying out studies comparing the distribution of stresses between different types of materials used for implant-supported crowns, which is why this research comparing these types of materials was carried out. In the present study, the performance of the three materials on implants was analysed and compared, obtaining individual results for each component, in which the DL model showed the highest values for the crown, 28.45 MPa, followed by the CP model with average values and the lowest values for the RN, in line with the results of the work by Chen et al. (2014) who obtained higher results for lithium disilicate in the in silico analysis of nano-ceramic resin and lithium disilicate simulated on a test disc representing a crown with the characteristics of these materials superimposed on a support ring and subjected to a loading sphere for stress distribution analysis. However, the aforementioned authors elucidated the performance of these materials in implant-supported rehabilitations, evaluating only the biomechanics of the prosthetic crown. With a view to a clinical projection, the current study analysed the stress distribution of these materials on abutments, implants and bone tissues, with the highest stress values for RN, being 14.89 MPa for cortical bone and 5.45 MPa for medullary bone, 57.66 MPa for implants and 65.53 MPa for abutments, followed by CP results, and with the lowest DL values.

Menini et al. (2013) in their research into the shock absorption capacity of restorative materials for prostheses on implants, following the methodology of a machine simulating human chewing, characterised that different restorative materials significantly affect the transmission of stress to the peri-implant bone, where the more elastic the materials, the lower the stress found. They also pointed out that, according to Hooke's law, the higher the modulus of elasticity of the material, the less the material will deform under pressure and the more the force will probably be transferred through the material. On the other hand, the more resilient the material, the more easily it will deform under pressure, i.e. the harder and stiffer the material, the greater the force transmitted to the implant. Rosentritt et al. (2017) complemented this by citing materials with a lower modulus of elasticity as an alternative for implant-supported restorations, due to their high stability and cushioning effects, in line with the hypothesis of the current research.

However, the results obtained refuted this hypothesis, since the hybrid materials, with greater resilience, obtained greater results in terms of stress propagation in the abutment structures, implants and bone tissue, compared to the less resilient ceramic with a higher modulus of elasticity, which contrasts with the descriptions of various studies cited, such as Menini et al. (2013), Chen et al. (2014), Kok et al. (2015), who emphasised the use of these materials with lower modulus of elasticity values, justifying better performance in terms of stress distribution in posterior implant-supported rehabilitations.

In this study, it was observed that the medullary bone showed lower stress values than the cortical bone. In addition, the medullary bone is further away from the region of greatest stress and has a lower modulus of elasticity. However, the current study considered a general analysis of the distribution of stresses in the peri-implant region.

It should be emphasised here that due to the in silico design of this study having certain limitations that directly complicate comparison and translation to clinical situations, the results obtained were considerably heterogeneous to the results of the studies by Menini et al. (2013), Chen et al. (2014), Kok et al. (2015) and Rosentritt et al. (2016), in terms of the performance of the different materials analysed, with the RN model having the highest peri-implant stress results. Thus, the results provide valid information and reveal important concepts for monolithic restorative materials, especially on posterior implants, and are precepts for future clinical studies, which are necessary to confirm the results obtained.

CHAPTER 7

CONCLUSION

According to the results obtained in this study, it can be concluded that the crown material influences the distribution of stresses, with lithium disilicate showing the best biomechanical performance.

REFERENCES[1]

Aboushelib MN, Elsafi MH. Survival of resin infiltrated ceramics underinfluence of fatigue. Dent Mater. 2016 Apr;32(4):529-34.

Albero A, Pascual A, Camps I, Grau-Benitez M. Comparative characterisation of a novel cad-cam polymer-infiltrated-ceramic-network. J Clin Exp Dent. 2015 Oct 1;7(4):e495-500.

AL-Makramani BMA, Razak AAA, Abu-Hassan MI. Strength of a new All-Ceramic **restorative material "Turkom-Cera" compared to two other Alumina-Based** All- ceramic systems. Advances in ceramics - Characterisation, raw materials, processing, properties, degradation and healing. Intech. 2011 Aug;14:260-80.

Alshehri SA. An investigation into the role of core porcelain thickness and lamination in determining the flexural strength of in-ceram dental materials. J Prosthodont. 2011 June;20(4):261-6.

Amoroso AP, Ferreira MB, Torcato LB, Pellizer EP, Mazaro JVQ, Gennari Filho H. Dental ceramics: properties, indications and clinical considerations. Rev Odontol Araçatuba. 2012 Jul-Dec;33(2):19-25.

Awada A, Nathanson D. Mechanical properties of resin-ceramic CAD/CAM restorative materials. J Prosthetic Dentistry. 2015 Oct;114(4):587-593

Badawy R, El-Mowafy O, Tam LE. Fracture toughness of chairside CAD/CAM materials - Alternative loading approach for compact tension test. Dent Mater. 2016 July;32(7):847-52.

Bayraktar MB, Gultekin BA, Yalcin S, Mijiritsky E. Effect of crown to implant ratio and implant dimensions on priimplant stress of splinted implant-supported crowns: A finite element analysis. Implant Dent. 2013 Aug;22(4):406-13.

Beuer F, Schweiger J, Edelhoff D. Digital dentistry: an overview of recent developments for CAD/CAM generated restorations. Br Dent J. 2008 May 10;204(9):505-11.

Bindl A, Luthy H, Mormann WH. Strength and fracture pattern of monolithic CAD/CAM-generated posterior crowns. Dent Mater. 2006 Jan;22(1):29-36.

Bispo LB. Dental ceramics: advantages and limitations of zirconia. Rev Bras Odontol. 2015 Jan-Jun;72(1/2):24-9.

Blatt M, Butignon LE, Bonachela WC. Finite element analysis applied to implant dentistry - a new reality from the virtual to the real. Innov Implant J. 2006 Dec;1(2):53-62.

Bonfante EA, Suzuki M, Lorenzoni FC, Sena LA, Hirata R, Bonfante G et al. Probability of survival of implant-supported metal ceramic and CAD/CAM resin nanoceramic crowns. Dent Mater. 2015 Aug;31(8):e168-77.

---

[1] According to the Standardisation Manual for Dissertations and Theses of the Faculdade São Leopoldo Mandic in 2014, based on Vancouver style, and abbreviation of journal titles in accordance with Index Medicus.

Cekic-Nagas I, Ergum G, Elgimez F, Vallittu PK, Lassila LVJ. Micro-shear bond strength of different resin cements to ceramic/glass-polymer CAD-CAM block materials. J Prosthodont Res. 2016 Oct;60(4):265-73.

Chen C, Trindade FZ, Jager N, Kleverlaan CJ, Feilzer AJ. The fracture resistance of a CAD/CAM Resin Nano Ceramic (RNC) and a CAD ceramic at different thicknesses. Dent Mater. 2014 Sept;30(9):954-62.

Cruz M, Wassall T, Toledo EM, Barra LPS, Cruz S. Finite element stress analysis of dental prostheses supported by straight and angled implants. Int J Oral Maxillofac Implants. 2009 May-June;24(3):391-403.

Deany IL. Recent advances in ceramics for dentistry. Crit Rev Oral Biol Med. 1996;7(2):134-43.

Della Bona A, Corazza PH, Zhang Y. Characterisation of a polymer-infiltrated ceramic-network material. Dent Mater. 2014 May;30(5):564-9.

Dogan DO, Goler O, Mustaf B, Ozcan M, Eyuboglu GB, Ulgey M. Fracture Resistance of Molar Crowns Fabricated with Monolithic All-Ceramic CAD/CAM Materials Cemented on Titanium Abutments: An In Vitro Study. J Prosthodont. 2017 June;26(4):309-14.

El-Damanhoury HM, Haj-Ali RN, Platt JA. Fracture resistance and microleakage of endocrowns utilising three CAD-CAM blocks. Oper Dent. 2015 Mar-Apr;40(2):201-10.

Fasbinder DJ, Dennison JB, Heys D, Neiva G. A clinical evaluation of chairside lithium disilicate CAD/CAM crowns: A two-year report. J Am Dent Assoc. 2010 June;141 Suppl 2:10S-4S.

Garcia LFR, Consani S, Cruz PC, Pires de Souza FCP. Critical analysis of the history and development of dental ceramics. RGO Rev Gaúch Odontol. 2011 Jan-Jun;59:67-73.

Geng JP, Tan KBC, Liu G. Application of finite element analysis in implant dentistry: a review of the literature. J Prosthet Dent. 2001 June;85(6):585-98.

Giordano R. Materials for chairside CAD/CAM - produced restorations. J Am Dent Assoc. 2006 Sept;137 Suppl:14S-21S.

Gomes EA, Assunção WG, Rocha EP, Santos PH. Dental ceramics: the current state. Cerâmica. 2008;54(331):319-25.

Guerra CMF, Neves CAF, Almeida ECB, Valones MAA, Guimarães RP. Current state of dental ceramics. Int J Dent. 2007 Jul-Sep;6(3):90-5.

Gultekin BA, Gultekin P, Yalcin S. Application of finite element analysis in implant dentistry. InTech. 2012;2:21-54.

Joda T, Huber S, Burki A, Zysset P, Bragger U. Influence of Abutment Design on Stiffness, Strength, and Failure of Implant-Supported Monolithic Resin Nano Ceramic (RNC) Crowns. Clin Implant Dent Relat Res. 2015 Dec;17(6): 1200-7.

Kassem AS, Atta O, El-Mowafy O. Fatigue resistance and mcroleakage of CAD-CAM ceramic and composite molar crowns. J Prosthodont. 2012 Jan;21(1):28-32.

Kelly JR, Benetti P. Ceramic materials in dentistry: historical evolution and current practice. Aust Dent J. 2011 June;56 Suppll :84-96.

Kim JH, Lee S, Park JS, Ryu JJ. Fracture Load of Monolithic CAD/CAM Lithium Disilicate Ceramic Crowns and Veneered Zirconia Crowns as a Posterior Implant Restoration. Implant Dent. 2013 Feb;22(1):66-70.

Kitamura E, Stegaroiu R, Nomura S, Miyakawa O. Biomechanical aspects of marginal bone resorption around osseointegrated implants: considerations based on a three-dimensional finite element analysis. Clin Oral Implants Res. 2004 Aug;15(4):401-12.

Kok P, Kleverlaan CJ, Jager N, Kuijs R, Feilzer AJ. Mechanical performance of implant-supported posterior crowns. J Prosthet Dent. 2015 July;114(1):59-66.

Kramer N, Reinelt C, Richter G, Frankenberger R. Four-year clinical performance and marginal analysis of pressed glass ceramic inlays luted with ormocer restorative vs. conventional luting composite. J Dent. 2009 Nov;37(11):813-9.

Lee KS, Shin JH, Kim JE, Kim JH, Lee WC, Shin SW et al. Biomechanical Evaluation of a Tooth Restored with High Performance Polymer PEKK Post-Core System: A 3D Finite Element Analysis. Biomed Res Int. 2017:137-127.

Lim K, Yap AU, Agarwalla SV, Tan KB, Rosa V. Reliability, failure probability, and strength of resin-based materials for CAD/CAM restorations. J Appl Oral Sci. 2016 Sep-Oct;24(5):447-52.

Lotti RS, Machado AW, Mazzieiro ET, Júnior JL. Scientific applicability of the finite element method. Rev Dental Press Ortodon Ortopedi Facial. 2006 Mar-Apr;11(2):35-43.

Macedo JP, Pereira J, Faria J, Pereira CA, Alves JL, Henriques B et al. Finite element analysis of stress extent at peri-implant boné surrounding external hexagon or Morse taper implants. J Mech Behav Biomed Mater. 2017 July;71:441-7.

Magne P, Schlishting LH, Maia HP, Baratieri LN. In vitro fatigue resistance of CAD/CAM composite resin and ceramic posterior occlusal veneers. J Prosthet Dent. 2010 Sept;104(3):149-57.

Maminskas J, Puisys A, Kuoppala R, Raustia A, Juodzbalys G. The Prosthetic Influence and Biomechanics on Peri-Implant Strain: a Systematic Literature Review of Finite Element Studies. J Oral Maxillofac Res. 2016 Sept 9;7(3):e4.

Marson FC, Manetti LP, Silva CO, Progiante PS, Takeshita WM. Longitudinal evaluation of metal-free crowns. BJSCR. 2013 Feb;1(1):11-7.

Mattei FP, Alexandre P, Chain MC. State of the art of ceramics in dentistry. Dent Sci. 2011;2(5):84-91.

Menini M, Conserva E, Tealdo T, Bevilacqua M, Pera F, Signori A et al. Shock Absorption Capacity of Restorative Materials for Dental Implant Prostheses: An In Vitro Study. Int J Prosthodont. 2013 Nov-Dec;26(6):549-56.

Merz BR, Hunenbart S, Belser UC. Mechanics of the Implant-Abutment Connection: An 8-Degree Taper Compared to a Butt Joint Connection. Int J Oral Maxillofac Implants. 2000 July-Aug;15(4):519-26.

Mesquita VT, Vasques EL. Multidisciplinary clinical management of aesthetic rehabilitation using pure ceramics. Rev Baiana Odontol. 2016 June;7(2):172-9.

Moraes SLD, Verri FR, Junior JFS, Almeida DAF, Mello CC, Pellizzer EP. A 3-D Finite Element Study of the Influence of Crown-Implant Ratio on Stress Distribution. Braz Dent J. 2013 Nov-Dec;24(6):635-41.

Otto T, Schneider D. Long-Term Clinical Results of Chairside Cerec CAD/CAM Inlays and Onlays: A Case Series. Int J Prosthodont. 2008 Jan-Feb;21(1):53-9.

Pita MS, Anchieta RB, Ribeiro AB, Pita DS, Zuim PRJ, Pellizzer EP. Fundamentals of occlusion in implant dentistry: Clinical guidelines and their prosthetic and biomechanical determinants. Rev Odontol Araçatuba. 2008 jan-jun;29(1):53-9.

Poticny DF, Klim J. CAD/CAM in-office technology: Innovations after 25 years for predictable, aesthetic outcomes. J Am Dent Assoc. 2010 June;141 Suppl2:5S-9S.

Renzetti PF, Mantovani MB, Corrêa GO, Michida SMA, Silva CO, Marson FC. Aesthetic anterior rehabilitation with metal-free crowns: clinical case report. Braz J Surg Clin Res. 2013 Sep-Nov;4(3):16-20.

Rolim RMA, Sarmento HR, Branco ACL, Campos F, Pereira SMB, Souza ROA. Clinical performance of metal-free ceramic restorations: Literature review. Rev Bras Ciênc Saúde. 2013;17(2):309-18.

Rosentritt M, Hahnel S, Engelhardt F, Behr M, Preis V. In vitro performance and fracture resistance of CAD/CAM-fabricated implant supported molar crowns. Clin Oral Investig. 2017 May;21(4):1213-9.

Silva MG. Influence of splinting of fixed prosthetic restorations and the number of implants on stress distribution in a posterior edentulous mandible [dissertation]. São Paulo: University of São Paulo; 2005.

Silva NRFA, Bonfante EA, Martins LM, Valverde GB, Thompson VP, Ferencz JL et al. Reliability of Reduced-thickness and Thinly Veneered Lithium Disilicate Crowns. J Dent Res. 2012 Mar;91(3):305-10.

Skalak R. Biomechanical considerations in osseointegrated prostheses. J Prosthet Dent. 1983 June;49(6):843-8.

Takahashi JMFK. Three-dimensional finite element analysis of the biomechanics of implant-supported prostheses: influence of occlusal load, connection type, implant angulation and modelling simplifications [thesis]. Piracicaba: Unicamp; 2011.

Tinschert J, Zweza D, Marxa R, Anusaviceb KJ. Structural reliability of alumina-, feldspar-, leucite-, mica- and zirconia-based ceramics. J Dent. 2000 Sept;28(7):529- 35.

Trivedi S. Finite element analysis: A boon to dentistry. J Oral Biol Craniofac Res. 2014 Sept-Dec;4(3):200-3.

Weyhrauch M, Igiel C, Scheller H, Weibrich G, Lehmann KM. Fracture Strength of Monolithic All-Ceramic Crowns on Titanium Implant Abutments. Int J Oral Maxillofac Implants. 2016 Mar-Apr;31(2):304-9.

Zandinejad A, Metz M, Stevens P, Lin W, Morton D. Virtually designed and CAD/CAM-fabricated lithium disilicate prostheses for an aesthetic maxillary rehabilitation: A senior dental student clinic report. J Prosthet Dent. 2015 Apr;113(4):282-8.

Zhi L, Bortolotto T, Krejci I. Comparative in vitro wear resistance of CAD/CAM composite resin and ceramic materials. J Prosthet Dent. 2016 Feb;115(2): 199-202.

ANNEX A - OPINION OF THE ETHICS COMMITTEE

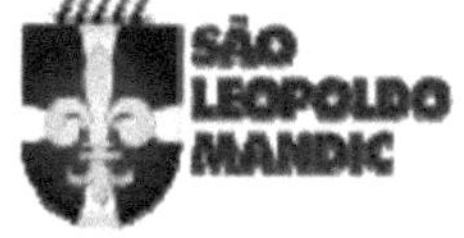

São Leopoldo Mandic
Centro de Pesquisas Odontológicas
Comunicado de Dispensa de Submissão ao Comitê

Campinas, 07 de maio de 2015

Prezado(a) Aluno(a): Gulbson da Silva Litaiff

O projeto abaixo descrito, apresentado ao respectivo Comitê de Ética, nesta Instituição, foi dispensado de ser submetido à análise, por tratar-se exclusivamente de pesquisa laboratorial. Sem envolvimento de seres humanos ou materiais.

Número do Protocolo: 2015/0464
Data da entrega do Projeto: 05/05/2015
Data da Reunião do Comitê: 25/05/2015

Orientado pelo(a) Prof(a) Dr(a): Milton Edson Miranda

Projeto: AVALIAÇÃO DO SISTEMA "SISTEMAS LAVA" ULTIMANTE 3M ESPE E IPS E.MAX (CAD/CAM) EM COROAS UNITÁRIAS IMPLANTO-SUPORTADAS: ANÁLISE TRIDIMENSIONAL DE ELEMENTOS FINITOS.

Cordialmente,

Profa. Dra. Fernanda Lopes da Cunha
Presidente do Comitê de Ética em Pesquisa

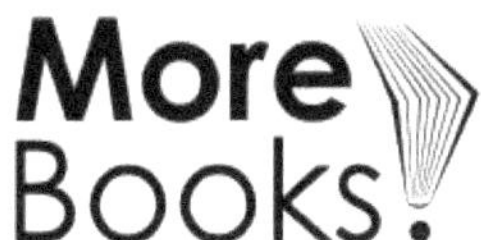

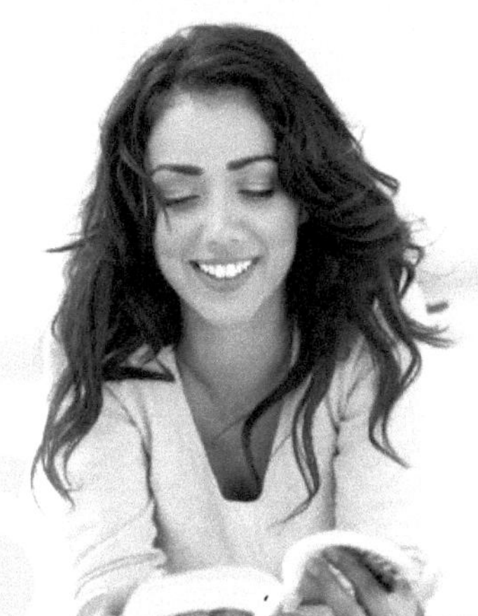

I want morebooks!

Buy your books fast and straightforward online - at one of world's fastest growing online book stores! Environmentally sound due to Print-on-Demand technologies.

Buy your books online at
www.morebooks.shop

Kaufen Sie Ihre Bücher schnell und unkompliziert online – auf einer der am schnellsten wachsenden Buchhandelsplattformen weltweit! Dank Print-On-Demand umwelt- und ressourcenschonend produziert.

Bücher schneller online kaufen
www.morebooks.shop

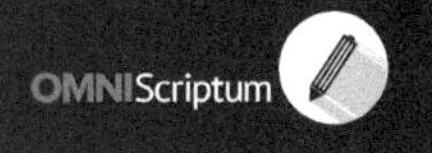